CW00450119

Veggie Treats

A Complete, Step-by-Step Cooking Guide for Your Homemade Vegetarian Desserts

Kaylee Collins

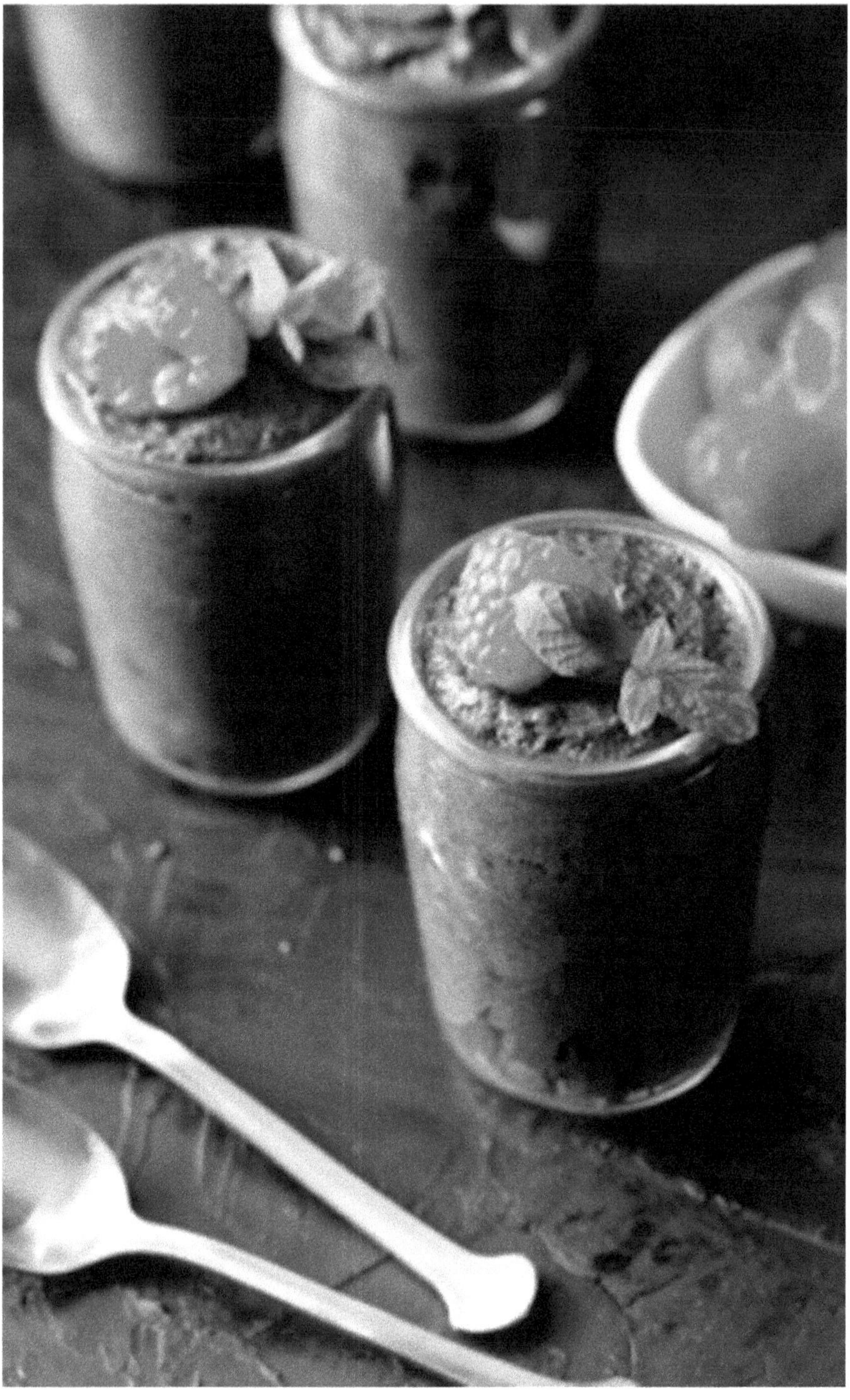

© Copyright 2021 - All rights reserved.

The content contained within this book may not be reproduced, duplicated or transmitted without direct written permission from the author or the publisher.

Under no circumstances will any blame or legal responsibility be held against the publisher, or author, for any damages, reparation, or monetary loss due to the information contained within this book. Either directly or indirectly.

Legal Notice:

This book is copyright protected. This book is only for personal use. You cannot amend, distribute, sell, use, quote or paraphrase any part, or the content within this book, without the consent of the author or publisher.

Disclaimer Notice:

Please note the information contained within this document is for educational and entertainment purposes only. All effort has been executed to present accurate, up to date, and reliable, complete information. No warranties of any kind are declared or implied. Readers acknowledge that the author is not engaging in the rendering of legal, financial, medical or professional advice. The content within this book has been derived from various sources. Please consult a licensed professional before attempting any techniques outlined in this book.

By reading this document, the reader agrees that under no circumstances is the author responsible for any losses, direct or indirect, which are incurred as a result of the use of information contained within this document, including, but not limited to, — errors, omissions, or inaccuracies.

Table of Contents

Blueberry-Peach Cobbler

(Prep time: 20 min| Cooking Time: 60 min | serve: 2)

Ingredients

5 peaches, peeled, pitted, and sliced

2 tablespoons fresh lemon juice

1 cup coconut sugar, divided

Pinch salt,

2 cups coconut flour, divided

1 teaspoon baking powder

½ cup coconut oil,

2 large eggs

1 teaspoon vanilla extract

1 cup buttermilk

2 cups fresh blueberries

Instructions

Place peaches in a large bowl. Drizzle with lemon juice; toss. Add coconut sugar, 1/8 teaspoon salt, and 2 tablespoons coconut flour to peach mixture; toss to combine. Arrange peach mixture evenly in a 8inch glass or baking dish coated with cooking spray.

Combine reaming coconut flour, remaining ¼ teaspoon salt, and baking powder in a bowl, stirring well with a whisk. Place the remaining coconut sugar and coconut oil in a medium bowl, and beat with a mixer at medium speed until light and fluffy (about 2 minutes). Add egg, 1 at a time, beating well after each addition. Stir in vanilla extract. Add flour mixture and buttermilk, beating just until combined. Stir in blueberries.

Spread batter evenly over peach mixture;

Pour 1 cup filtered water into the Instant Pot and insert the trivet.

Using a sling if desired, place the pan onto the trivet, Close the lid, set the pressure release to sealing, and select Manual/Pressure Cook. Set the Instant Pot to 55 minutes on High pressure, and Once cooked, let the pressure naturally disperse from the Instant Pot for about 10 minutes, then carefully switch the pressure release to Venting.

Nutrition Facts

Calories 346, Total Fat 18.6g, Saturated Fat 14.4g, Cholesterol 48mg, Sodium 76mg, Total Carbohydrate 38.4g, Dietary Fiber 14.4g, Total Sugars 14.1g, Protein 7.9g

Coconut-Blackberries Flaxseed Pudding

Prep time: 10 min Cooking Time: 05 min serve: 2

Ingredients

½ cup almond milk

½ cup Water

½ cup blackberries

½ cup flex seeds

½ cup quinoa

1/8 cup honey

¼ teaspoon pure vanilla extract

Fresh berries for garnish

Instructions

Combine the almond milk, water, blackberries, flex seeds, quinoa, honey, and vanilla extract in the inner pot.

Lock the lid into place. Select Pressure Cook or Manual; set the pressure to High and the time to 3 minutes. Make sure the steam release knob is in the sealed position. After cooking, naturally release the pressure for 5 minutes, then quick release any remaining pressure.

Unlock and remove the lid. Pour the pudding into individual serving cups and refrigerate until it sets, about 1 hour.

Serve cold garnished with blackberries.

Nutrition Facts

Calories 454, Total Fat 22.1g, Saturated Fat 13g, Cholesterol 0mg , Sodium 44mg, Total Carbohydrate 46.3g, Dietary Fiber 14.2g, Total Sugars 6g, Protein 17.9g

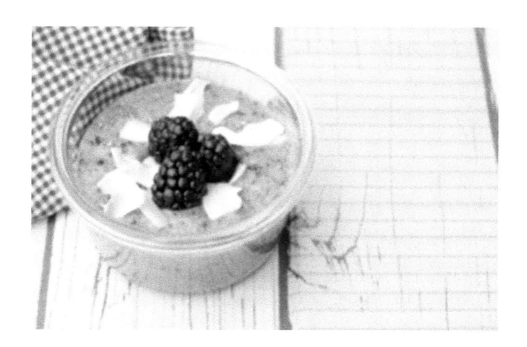

Baked Quinoa

Prep time: 10 min Cooking Time: 70 min serve: 2

Ingredients

½ tablespoon avocado oil

½ tablespoon honey

1 egg

1 tablespoon almond butter

¼ cup coconut milk

¼ teaspoon Vanilla

½ cup Quinoa

¼ teaspoon baking powder

Pinch salt

1/8 cup chocolate chips

Powdered sugar for garnish

Instructions

In a medium bowl, beat together avocado oil and honey. Add egg a time and beat until uniform.

Add almond butter, coconut milk and vanilla and stir to combine.

In a large bowl, stir together quinoa, baking powder and salt. Add wet Ingredients and mix until fully incorporated.

Fold in chocolate chips.

Coat the inside of a 7-inch baking pan or casserole with non-stick spray-

Spread batter in pan and cover pan with foil.

Pour one cup of water in the Instant Pot and insert the steam rack. Lower the pan or casserole on to the steam rack, secure the lid, and make sure the vent is closed.

Use the display panel to select the Manual or Pressure Cook function. Use the + /- keys and program the Instant Pot for 45 minutes.

When the time is up, let the pressure naturally release for 15 minutes, quickly releasing the remaining pressure.

Carefully remove the pan and allow to cool for 10 minutes before serving.

Garnish with powdered sugar (optional). Keep covered and serve

Nutrition Facts

Calories 392, Total Fat 20g, Saturated Fat 9.9g, Cholesterol 84mg, Sodium 125mg, Total Carbohydrate

41.7g, Dietary Fiber 5g, Total Sugars 11.3g, Protein 12g

Rich Antioxidant Cheesecake

Prep time:15 min Cooking Time: 25 min serve: 2

Ingredients

Base

½ cup feta cheese softened

1-1/2 teaspoon coconut flour

1-1/2 tablespoons coconut cream

1 egg

½ tablespoon moringa powder

¼ teaspoon vanilla extract

Topping

1/8 cup brown sugar

1/2 cup coconut cream

Instructions

Combine the feta cheese, coconut flour, coconut cream, egg, moringa powder, and vanilla in a large bowl. Mix thoroughly. Place mixture in spring form pan, then loosely cover with aluminium foil. 2. Pour 2 cups filtered water into Instant Pot, then add trivet, placing the spring form pan atop the rack.

Move the valve to Sealing and close the lid of the Instant Pot.

Set to Manual/Pressure Cook, and let cook for 25 minutes at High pressure. Once cooked, let the pressure naturally disperse from the Instant Pot for about 10 minutes, then carefully switch the pressure release to Venting.

Remove pan, and let cool for 30 minutes. Then refrigerate for at least 45 minutes (a few hours is preferable).

Remove foil. Mix the brown sugar and coconut cream in a small bowl, spread evenly on the cake before serving. Store any remaining cheesecake in the refrigerator.

Nutrition Facts

Calories 192, Total Fat 12.1g, Saturated Fat 8g, Cholesterol 115mg, Sodium 456mg, Total Carbohydrate 13.2g, Dietary Fiber 0.9g , Total Sugars 10.8g, Protein 8.7g

Lemon curd & blueberry loaf cake

Prep: 20 mins Cook:1 hr and 15 mins easy Cuts into 8-10 slices

Ingredients

175g softened butter

500ml tub Greek yogurt (you need 100ml/3.5fl oz in the cake, the rest to serve)

300g jar good lemon curd (you need 2 tbsp in the cake, the rest to serve)

3 eggs zest and juice 1 lemon, plus extra zest to serve

200g self-raising flour 175g golden caster sugar

200g punnet of blueberries (you need 85g/3oz in the cake, the rest to serve) 140g icing sugar

edible flowers, such as purple or yellow primroses, to serve (optional)

Directions:

1 Heat oven to 160C/140C fan/gas 3. Grease a 2lb loaf tin and line with a long strip of baking parchment. Put 100g yogurt, 2 tbsp lemon curd, the softened butter, eggs, lemon zest, flour and caster sugar into a large mixing bowl. Quickly mix with an electric whisk until the batter just comes together. Scrape half into the prepared tin. Weigh 85g blueberries from the punnet

and sprinkle half into the tin, scrape the rest of the batter on top, then scatter the other half of the 85g berries. Bake for 1 hr 10 mins-1 hr 15 mins until golden, and a skewer poked into the centre comes out clean. 2 Cool in the tin, then carefully lift onto a serving plate to ice. Sift the icing sugar into a bowl and stir in enough lemon juice to make a thick, smooth icing. Spread

over the top of the cake, then decorate with lemon zest and edible flowers, if you like. Serve in slices with extra lemon curd, Greek yogurt and blueberries.

Winter wonderland cake

Prep:1 hr Cook:35 mins Plus cooling easy Serves 12

Ingredients

175g unsalted butter, softened, plus more for the tin 250g golden caster sugar

3 large eggs

225g plain flour

2 tsp baking powder 50g crème fraîche

100g dark chocolate, melted and cooled a little

3 tbsp strawberry jam

8-10 candy canes, red and white mini white meringues and jelly sweets, to decorate

For the angel frosting

500g white caster sugar

1 tsp vanilla extract 1 tbsp liquid glucose

2 egg whites 30g icing sugar, sifted

Directions:

Heat oven to 180C/160C fan/gas 4. Butter and line three 18cm (or two 20cm) cake tins. Beat the butter and sugar together until light and fluffy. Add the eggs, beating them in one at a time. Fold in the flour, baking powder and a pinch of salt, fold in the crème fraîche and chocolate and 100ml boiling water. 2 Divide the cake mixture between the tins and level the tops the batter. Bake for 25-30 mins or until a skewer inserted into the middle comes out clean. Leave to cool for 10 mins in the tin, then tip out onto a cooling rack and peel off the parchment. Set aside to cool completely. 3 To make the angel frosting, put the sugar, vanilla and liquid glucose in a pan with 125ml water. Bring to the boil and cook until the sugar has melted – the syrup turns transparent and the mixture hits 130C on a sugar thermometer (be very careful with hot sugar). Take off the heat.

Meanwhile, beat the egg whites until stiff then, while still beating, gradually pour in the hot sugar syrup in a steady stream. Keep beating until the mixture is fluffy and thick enough to spread – this might take a few mins as the mixture cools. Beat in the icing sugar. 4 Spread two of the sponges with jam and some of the icing mixture, then sandwich the cakes together with the plain one on top. Use a little of the frosting to ice the whole cake (don't worry about crumbs at this stage). Use the remaining icing to ice the cake again, smoothing the side, and swirling it on top. Crush four of the candy canes and sprinkle over the cake, then add the remaining whole candy canes, meringues and sweets.

Nutty cinnamon & yogurt dipper

Prep:5 mins No cook easy Serves 1

Ingredients

100g natural Greek yogurt

1 tbsp nut butter (try almond or cashew)

¼ tsp ground cinnamon 1 tsp honey To serve

apple wedges (tossed in a little lemon juice to prevent them turning brown)

celery sticks

carrot sticks

mini rice cakes or crackers (choose gluten-free brands if necessary)

Directions:

1 In a small tub, mix the yogurt, nut butter, cinnamon and honey. Serve with apple wedges (tossed in a little lemon juice to prevent them turning brown), celery or carrot sticks, and mini rice cakes or crackers.

Coconut bauble truffles

Prep:45 mins plus at least 2 hrs chilling, no cook Easy Makes about 25

Ingredients

250g madeira cake

85g ready-to-eat dried apricots, finely chopped

25g desiccated coconut

125ml light condensed milk To decorate

140g desiccated coconut

different food colourings, we used yellow, pink, blue and purple

Directions:

In a big mixing bowl, crumble the cake with your fingers – try to get the bits as small as possible.

Tip in the apricots and coconut. Using your hands again, mix with the cake crumbs. Use a wooden spoon to stir in the condensed milk. After you've mixed it in a bit, use your fingers to pull off any bits stuck to the spoon. Squidge everything together with your hands until it is well mixed and all the cake crumbs are sticky. Rub your hands together over the bowl so any bits that are stuck drop off.

Line some trays that fit in your fridge with baking parchment. Roll the sticky cake mixture into small balls (about the size of a conker or gobstopper) between your hands. Line them up on the trays, then put them in the fridge while you get the decorations ready.

Decide how many different food colorings you will use, then split the coconut into the same number of piles. Put each pile of coconut into a plastic sandwich bag, add a few drops of food colouring to each, and tie a knot in the top. Shake the bags and scrunch between your fingers until all the coconut is coloured – if it's not bright enough, open the bag and add a few more drops of colouring.

Open all the bags of coloured coconut and take the truffles from the fridge. Put 1 tbsp of water in a small bowl and lightly coat each truffle in it so the coconut can stick to the outside of each bauble.

One by one, drop each truffle into one of your bags. Shake it and roll it around until the outside is covered in coconut. Carefully put each truffle back onto the trays and chill for at least another 2 hrs until they are freezing.

If you like, put some of the truffles in gift bags or boxes and tie with ribbons to give as presents. Will keep in the fridge for up to 1 week.

Christmas cake cupcakes

Prep:40 mins Cook:45 mins easy Makes 12

Ingredients

For the batter

200g dark muscovado sugar

175g butter

700g luxury mixed dried fruit

50g glacé cherries

2 tsp grated fresh root ginger zest and juice

1 orange

100ml dark rum, brandy or orange juice

85g/3oz pecan nuts, roughly chopped

3 large eggs, beaten

85g ground almond

200g plain flour ½ tsp baking powder

1 tsp mixed spice

1 tsp cinnamon For the icing

400g pack ready-rolled marzipan (we used Dr Oetker)

4 tbsp warm apricot jam or shredless marmalade

500g pack fondant icing sugar

icing sugar, for dusting

6 gold and 6 silver muffin cases 6 gold and 6 silver sugared almond

snowflake sprinkles

Directions:

Tip the sugar, butter, dried fruit, whole cherries, ginger, orange zest and juice into a large pan. Pour over the rum, brandy or juice, then put on the heat and slowly bring to the boil, stirring frequently to melt the butter. Reduce the heat and bubble gently, uncovered for 10 mins, stirring now and again to make sure the mixture doesn't catch on the bottom of the pan. Set aside for 30 mins to cool.

Stir the nuts, eggs and ground almonds into the fruit, then sift in the flour, baking powder and spices. Stir everything together gently but thoroughly. Your batter is ready. Heat oven to 150C/130C fan/gas 2.

Scoop the cake mix into 12 deep muffin cases (an ice-cream scoop works well), then level tops with a spoon dipped in hot water. Bake for 35-45 mins until golden and just firm to touch. A skewer inserted should come out clean. Cool on a wire rack.

Unravel the marzipan onto a work surface lightly dusted with icing sugar. Stamp out 12 rounds, 6cm across. Brush the cake tops with apricot jam, top with a marzipan round and press down lightly.Make up the fondant icing to a spreading consistency, then swirl on top of each cupcake. Decorate with sugared almonds and snowflakes, then leave to set. Will keep in a tin for 3 weeks.

Fruity ice-lolly pens

Prep:10 mins Cook:15 mins - 20 mins Easy Makes 6

Ingredients

50ml sugar-free blackcurrant cordial

50ml sugar-free orange cordial

5 tsp each red and orange natural food colouring, plus extra for painting

50g blueberry

50g strawberry, chopped

a few red grapes, halved

Directions:

Pour each cordial into a separate jug, and add the corresponding food colouring. Stir in 100ml water.

Put the blueberries, strawberries and grapes into the ice-lolly moulds and pour the blackcurrant mixture up to the brim of 3 moulds.

Pour the orange cordial into the remaining 3 moulds. Freeze for 4 hrs. 2Remove the lollies from the moulds and dot extra food colouring onto a dish.

Dip the lollies into the colouring and use to draw on clean paper– while enjoying the lolly at the same time.

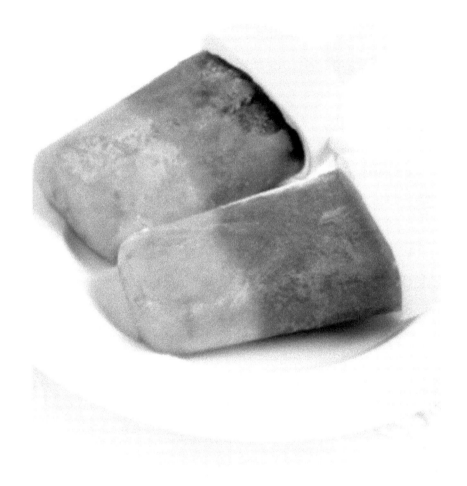

Chocolate & raspberry pots

Prep:15 mins Cook:10 mins Serves 6

Ingredients

200g plain chocolate (not too bitter, 50% or less)

100g frozen raspberry, defrosted or fresh raspberries 500g Greek yogurt

3 tbsp honey

chocolate curls or sprinkles, for serving

Directions:

Break the chocolate into small pieces and place in a heatproof bowl. Bring a little water to the boil in a small saucepan, then place the bowl of chocolate on top, making sure the bottom of the bowl does not touch the water. Leave the chocolate to melt slowly over a low heat.

Remove the chocolate from the heat and leave to cool for 10 mins. Meanwhile, divide the raspberries between 6 small ramekins or glasses.

When the chocolate has cooled slightly, quickly mix in the yogurt and honey. Spoon the chocolate mixture over the raspberries. Place in the fridge to cool, then finish the pots with a few chocolate shavings before serving.

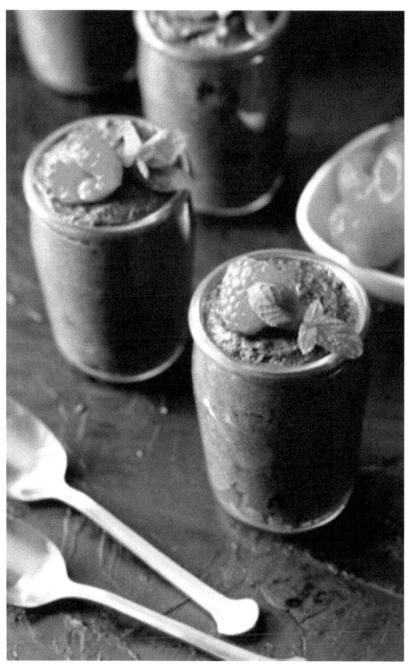

Vegan Black Bean Brownies

These easy Vegan Black Bean Brownies are a healthy chocolate dessert, low- calorie, low-carb and gluten-free with no added sugar, only 5 grams of net carbs per serve.

Prep Time: 10 mins Cook Time: 25 mins Total Time: 35 mins

Ingredients

Black Bean Brownies

1/4 cup Coconut oil + 1 teaspoon to grease pan

3.5 oz Sugar-free Dark Chocolate - see note for details 1 can Black beans , rinsed, drained (15 oz)

1 cup Almond Flour

3/4 cup Unsweetened apple sauce

1 teaspoon Baking Powder Caramelized Pecan

1 teasponn Coconut oil

1/4 cup peacan roughly chopped

2 tablespoon Sugar-free flavored maple syrup Dark Chocolate Drizzle

1 oz Sugar-free Dark Chocolate , melted, - see note for options

Black Bean Brownies

Instructions

Preheat oven to 300F (150C).

Line an 8 inches x 8 inches square brownie pan with parchment paper. Rub a little coconut oil on it to make sure it does not stick. Set aside.

In a small mixing bowl, add dark chocolate and coconut oil, microwave by 30-second bursts, stir and repeat until fully melted. If you don't have a microwave use a saucepan and melt under low heat until fully melted. Set aside.

In a food processor, with the S blade attachment, add all the ingredients: melted oil/chocolate mixture, black beans, baking powder, almond meal unsweetened applesauce

Pour into the prepared pan and spread evenly. Bake for 25-30 minutes max.

Cool down 5 minutes in the pan then lift out the parchment paper to unmold the brownie.

Place the brownie on a rack, drizzle extra melted chocolate on top if you like. I melted my chocolate in a small bowl in the microwave. Go with 30-second burst, stir, repeat until melted and drizzle over the brownie!

Caramelized Pecan Nuts

Melt coconut oil in a small frying pan over low heat.

Add roughly chopped pecan nuts and maple syrup.

Cook for 2 to 3 minutes, stirring constantly until it caramelizes. Spread out on parchment paper to cool.

Sprinkle over the brownie after drizzling the melted chocolate. This brownie is getting super fudgy when stored in the fridge. I recommend to store in an airtight plastic box in the fridge up to 3 days or in a cookie jar in the pantry.

Chocolate options: You can use any chocolate in this recipe. I tested 70% cocoa dark chocolate which gives the perfect sweetness, it's sugar-free and it gives a perfectly sweet brownie without the extra carbs or sugar (get Sugar Free Lillys Bars here affiliate link). You can also use 85% cocoa chocolate for a bitter/less sweet brownie.

Sugar free/low carb: don't use maple syrup to caramelize the nuts. Use same amount of sugar free crystal sweetener like swerve.

Nutrition Info

Fat 7.3g11% Carbohydrates 8.7g3% Fiber 3.5g15%

Sugar 1.3g1% Protein 3.2g6% Net Carbs 5.2g

Simple nutty pancakes

Prep: 5 mins Cook:5 mins easy makes 4

Ingredients

150g self-raising flour

½ tsp baking powder

1 large egg 150ml milk

2 tbsp agave syrup, plus extra to serve

50 g mixed nuts, chopped

2 tbsp rapeseed oil, for frying

Directions:

Tip the flour and baking powder into a large bowl with a pinch of salt. Make a well in the centre, then add the egg, milk and syrup. Whisk until smooth, then fold in half the nuts.

Heat 1 tbsp oil in a large, non-stick frying pan over a medium-high heat. Spoon two ladles of the mixture into the pan and cook for 1 min each side. Repeat to make two more.

Serve with a drizzle of agave syrup and the remaining nuts for extra crunch.

Flowerpot chocolate chip muffins

Prep: 10 mins Cook:12 mins - 15 mins Easy Makes 10 mini-muffins

Ingredients

3 tbsp vegetable oil

125g plain flour

1 tsp baking powder

25g cocoa powder

100g golden caster sugar

1 large egg 100ml milk 150g milk chocolate chips

25g chocolate cake decorations such as vermicelli sprinkles or chocolate-coated popping candy

20 rice paper wafer daisies (these come in packs of 12, so get 2 packs)

10 mini teracotta pots

Directions:

Heat oven to 180C/160C fan/gas 4. Lightly oil the inside of the terracotta pots with a little vegetable oil and place on a baking tray. Place a paper mini muffin case in the bottom of each pot.

Put the flour, baking powder and cocoa in a bowl and stir in the sugar.

Crack the egg into a jug and whisk with the milk and remaining oil. Pour this over the flour and cocoa mixture, and stir in with 50g of the chocolate chips. Be careful not to overmix – you want a loose but still quite lumpy mixture. Spoon into the pots up to three- quarters complete. Place in the middle of the oven and bake for 12-15 mins until risen and firm. Transfer to a wire rack (still in the pots) and leave to cool.

Put the rest of the chocolate chips in a small bowl and melt over a small pan of gently simmering water (don't let the water touch the bowl), or put in a microwave-proof bowl and heat on High for 1 min until melted.

Spread the tops of the muffins with the melted chocolate. Sprinkle over the chocolate decorations and add 2 rice paper wafer daisies to each pot to serve. Will keep for 2 days in an airtight container.

Sticky plum flapjack bars

Prep:20 mins Cook:1 hr Easy Makes 18

Ingredients

450g fresh plum, halved, stoned and roughly sliced

½ tsp mixed spice

300g light muscovado sugar

350g butter

300g rolled porridge oats (not jumbo)

140g plain flour

50g chopped walnut pieces

3 tbsp golden syrup

Directions:

Heat oven to 200C/180C fan/gas 6. Tip the plums into a bowl. Toss with the spice, 50g of the sugar and a small pinch of salt, then set aside to macerate.

Gently melt the butter in a saucepan. In a large bowl, mix the oats, flour, walnut pieces and remaining sugar, making sure there are no lumps of sugar, then stir in the butter and golden syrup until everything is combined into a loose flapjack mixture.

Grease a square baking tin about 20 x 20cm. Press half the oaty mix over the base of the tin, then tip over the plums and spread to make an even layer. Press the remaining oats over the plums so they are entirely covered right to the sides of the tin. Bake for 45-50 mins until dark golden and starting to crisp a little around the edges. Leave to cool completely, then cut into 18 little bars. Will keep in an airtight container for 2 days or can be frozen for up to a month.

Easter chocolate bark

Prep: 20 mins Cook:5 mins plus cooling easy Makes enough for 6-8 gift bags

Ingredients

3 x 200g bars milk chocolate

2 x 90g packs mini chocolate eggs

1 heaped tsp freeze-dried raspberry pieces – or you could use crystallised petals

Directions:

Break the chocolate into a large heatproof bowl. Bring a pan of water to a simmer, then sit the bowl on top. The water must not touch the bottom of the bowl. Let the chocolate slowly melt, stirring now and again with a spatula. For best results, temper your chocolate (see tip).

Meanwhile, lightly grease then line a 23 x 33cm roasting tin or baking tray with parchment. Put three-quarters of the mini eggs into a food bag and bash them with a rolling pin until broken up a little.

When the chocolate is smooth, pour it into the tin. Tip the tin from side to side to let the chocolate find the corners and level out. Scatter with the smashed and whole mini eggs, followed by the freeze- dried raspberry pieces. Leave to set, then remove from the parchment and snap into shards, ready to pack in boxes or bags.

Chocolate fudge cupcakes

Prep:30 mins Cook:25 mins - 30 mins Plus cooling easy Makes 12

Ingredients

200g butter

200g plain chocolate, under 70% cocoa solids is fin 200g light, soft brown sugar

2 eggs, beaten

1 tsp vanilla extract

250g self-raising flour

Smarties, sweets and sprinkles, to decorate

For the icing

200g plain chocolate

100ml double cream, not fridge-cold

50g icing sugar

Directions:

Heat oven to 160C/140C fan/gas 3 and line a 12-hole muffin tin with cases. Gently melt the butter, chocolate, sugar and 100ml hot water together in a large saucepan, stirring occasionally, then set aside to cool a little while you weigh the other ingredients.

Stir the eggs and vanilla into the chocolate mixture. Put the flour into a large mixing bowl, then stir in the chocolate mixture until smooth. Spoon into cases until just over three- quarters full (you may have a little mixture leftover), then set aside for 5 mins before putting on a low shelf in the oven and baking for 20-22 mins. Leave to cool.

For the icing, melt the chocolate in a heatproof bowl over a pan of barely simmering water. Once melted, turn off the heat, stir in the double cream and sift in the icing sugar. When spreadable, top each cake with some and decorate with your favourite sprinkles and sweets.

Marshmallows dipped in chocolate

Prep: 10 mins Cook:5 mins Plus setting time easy Makes 26 approx

Ingredients

50g white chocolate

50g milk chocolate

selection of cake sprinkles

1 bag marshmallows (about 200g)

1 pack lollipop sticks

Directions:

Heat the chocolate in separate bowls over simmering water or on a low setting in the microwave. Allow to cool a little.

Put your chosen sprinkles on separate plates. Push a cake pop or lolly stick into a marshmallow about half way in. Dip into the white or milk chocolate, allow the excess to drip off then dip into the sprinkles of your choice. Put into a tall glass to set. Repeat with each marshmallow.

Christmas pudding Rice Krispie cakes

Prep: 30 hrs Cook:5 mins plus chilling Easy Makes 10 - 12

Ingredients

50g rice pops (we used Rice Krispies)

30g raisin, chopped

50g butter

100g milk chocolate, broken into pieces

2 tbsp crunchy peanut butter

30g mini marshmallow

80g white chocolate ready-made icing holly leaves

Directions:

Put the rice pops and raisins into a bowl. Put the butter, milk chocolate, peanut butter and marshmallows into a small saucepan. Place on a medium to low heat and stir until the chocolate and butter have melted but the marshmallows are just beginning to melt.

Pour onto the rice pops and stir until well coated. Line an egg cup with cling film. Press about a tablespoon of the mixture into the egg cup. Press firmly and then remove, peel off the cling film and place the pudding into a cake case, flat-side down. Repeat with the remaining mixture. Chill until firm.

Melt the white chocolate in the microwave or bowl over a saucepan of barely simmering water. Spoon a little chocolate over the top of each pudding. Top with icing holly leaves.

Yummy chocolate log

Prep:30 mins Cook:10 mins More effort Serves 8

Ingredients

For the cake

3 eggs

85g golden caster sugar

85g plain flour (minus 2 tbsp)

2 tbsp cocoa powder

½ tsp baking powder

For the filling & icing • 50g butter, plus extra for the tin

140g dark chocolate, broken into squares

1 tbsp golden syrup

284ml pot double cream

200g icing sugar, sifted

2-3 extra strong mints, crushed (optional)

icing sugar and holly sprigs to decorate - ensure you remove the berries before serving

Directions:

Heat the oven to 200C/180C fan/gas 6. Butter and line a 23 x 32cm Swiss roll tin with baking parchment. Beat the eggs and golden caster sugar together with an electric whisk for about 8 mins until thick and creamy. Mix the flour, cocoa powder and baking powder, then sift onto the egg mixture. Fold in very carefully, then pour into the tin. Tip the tin from side to side to spread the mixture into the corners. Bake for 10 mins.

Lay a sheet of baking parchment on a work surface. When the cake is ready, tip it onto the parchment, peel off the lining paper, then roll the cake up from its longest edge with the paper inside. Leave to cool.

To make the icing, melt the butter and dark chocolate together in a bowl over a pan of hot water. Take from the heat and stir in the golden syrup and 5 tbsp double cream. Beat in the icing sugar until smooth.

Whisk the remaining double cream until it holds its shape. Unravel the cake, spread the cream over the top, scatter over the crushed extra strong mints, if using, then carefully roll up again into a log.

Cut a thick diagonal slice from one end of the log. Lift the log on to a plate, then arrange the slice on the side with the diagonal cut against the cake to make a branch. Spread the icing over the log and branch (don't cover the ends), then use a fork to mark the icing to give tree bark effect. Scatter with unsifted icing sugar to resemble snow, and decorate with holly.

Easy Easter nests

Prep: 25 mins Cook:8 mins Plus chilling easy Makes 12

Ingredients

200g milk chocolate, broken into pieces

85g shredded wheat, crushed

2 x 100g bags mini chocolate eggs

cupcake cases

Directions:

Melt the chocolate in a small bowl placed over a pan of barely simmering water. Pour the chocolate over the shredded wheat and stir well to combine.

Spoon the chocolate wheat into 12 cupcake cases and press the back of a teaspoon in the centre to create a nest shape. Place 3 mini chocolate eggs on top of each nest. Chill the nests in the fridge for 2 hrs until set.

Choco-dipped tangerines

Prep: 10 mins Easy Serves 1

Ingredients

1 tangerine, peeled and segmented

10g dark chocolate, melted

Directions:

Dip half of each tangerine segment in the melted chocolate, then put on a baking sheet lined with parchment. Keep in the fridge for 1 hr to set completely, or overnight if you prefer.

Chocolate crunch bars

Cook: 5 mins Prep: 20 mins plus chilling Easy Cuts into 12

Ingredients

100g butter, roughly chopped

300g dark chocolate (such as Bournville), broken into squares

3 tbsp golden syrup

140g rich tea biscuit, roughly crushed

12 pink marshmallows, quartered (use scissors)

2 x 55g bars Turkish delight

Directions:

Gently melt the butter, chocolate and syrup in a pan over a low heat, stirring frequently until smooth, then cool for about 10 mins.

Stir the biscuits and sweets into the pan until well mixed, then pour into a 17cm square tin lined with foil and spread the mixture to level it roughly. Chill until stiff, then cut into fingers.

Fruity Neapolitan lolly loaf

Prep: 25 mins 25 mins plus 8 hours freezing time Easy Serves 8

Ingredients

200g peaches nectarines or apricots (or a mixture), stoned

200g strawberries or raspberries (or a mixture), hulled

450ml double cream

½ x 397g can condensed milk

2 tsp vanilla extract orange and pink food colouring (optional)

8 wooden lolly sticks

Directions:

Put the peaches, nectarines or apricots in a food processor and pulse until they're chopped and juicy but still with some texture. Scrape into a bowl. Repeat with the berries and scrape into another bowl.

Pour the cream, condensed milk and vanilla into a third bowl and whip until just holding soft peaks. Add roughly a third of the mixture to the peaches and another third to the berries, and mix until well combined. Add a drop of orange food colouring to the peach mixture and a drop of pink food colouring to the berry mixture if you want a vibrant colour. Line a 900g loaf tin or terrine mould with cling film (look for a long thin one, ours was

23 x 7 x 8cm), then pour in the berry mixture. Freeze for 2 hrs and chill the remaining mixtures in the fridge.

Once the bottom layer is frozen, remove the vanilla mixture from the fridge and pour over the berry layer. The bottom layer should now be firm enough to support your lolly sticks, so place these, evenly spaced, along the length of the loaf tin, pushing down gently until they stand up straight. Return to the freezer for another 2 hrs.

Once the vanilla layer is frozen, pour over the peach mixture, easing it around the lolly sticks. Return to the freezer for a further 4 hrs or until completely frozen. Remove from the freezer 10 mins before serving. Use the cling film to help you remove the loaf from the tin. Take to the table on a board and slice off individual lollies for your guests. Any leftovers can be kept in the freezer for up to 2 weeks.

Keto Breakfast Brownie Muffins

Servingss 6

Ingredients

1 cup golden flaxseed meal

¼ cup cocoa powder

1 tablespoon cinnamon

½ tablespoon baking powder

½ teaspoon salt 1 large egg

2 tablespoons coconut oil

¼ cup sugar-free caramel syrup

½ cup pumpkin puree

1 teaspoon vanilla extract

1 teaspoon apple cider vinegar

¼ cup slivered almonds

Instructions

Preheat your oven to 350°F and combine all your dry ingredients in a deep mixing bowl and mix to combine.

In a separate bowl, combine all your wet ingredients.

Pour your wet ingredients into your dry ingredients and mix very well to combine.

Line a muffin tin with paper liners and spoon about ¼ cup of batter into each muffin liner. This recipe should Servings 6 muffins. Then sprinkle slivered almonds over the top of each muffin and press gently so that they adhere.

Bake in the oven for about 15 minutes. You should see the muffins rise and set on top. Enjoy warm or cool!

Nutrition Info

193 Calories 14.09g Fats 4.37g Net Carbs 6.98g Protein.

Walnut Cardamom Bar Cookies

Prep time: 20 min Cooking Time: 30 min serve: 2

Ingredients

¼ tablespoon butter, softened

½ tablespoon honey

1 egg, separated

½ tablespoon vanilla extract

1 cup coconut flour

½ teaspoon cardamom

½ teaspoon salt

½ tablespoon chopped walnut

½ tablespoons Butter

¼ teaspoon vanilla extract

1 tablespoon coconut milk, or as needed

Instructions

Grease a pan.

In a large bowl, cream together 1cup of butter, honey and light and fluffy. Mix in the egg yolk and vanilla. Combine the coconut flour, cardamom and salt; stir into the batter until it forms a soft dough. Spread evenly in the prepared pan. Brush the top with egg white and sprinkle walnut over the top.

Pour the water into the Instant Pot Insert, and place a trivet with the covered brownie cake tin into the Instant Pot.

Cover your Instant Pot, set the vent to Sealing, select the Manual or pressure cook button, select high pressure and set the timer to 20 mins.

When done allow the pot to undergo natural pressure release for 15 mins

Nutrition Facts

Calories 155, Total Fat 7.7g, Saturated Fat 3.5g, Cholesterol 93mg, Sodium 644mg, Total Carbohydrate

20.5g, Dietary Fiber 0.3g , Total Sugars 19.7g, Protein 3.4g

Lemon-Lime Magic Cake

Prep time: 20 min Cooking Time: 40 min serve: 2

Ingredients

Cake Layer

½ cup almond flour

1 cup coconut milk

½ cup butter melted

2 eggs

Lemon-Lime Layer

2 eggs, slightly beaten

1 tablespoon honey

1 tablespoon finely grated lemon peel

1 tablespoon finely grated lime peel

¼ tablespoon fresh lemon juice

¼ tablespoon fresh lime juice

Topping

1 container (4 Oz) Cool Whip frozen whipped topping, thawed

Instructions

Cake Layer:

In large bowl, beat almond flour, coconut milk, butter and eggs with electric mixer on medium speed 2 minutes, scraping bowl occasionally. Pour in pan. 3. Lemon-Lime Layer: In another large bowl, mix eggs, honey, lemon peel, lemon juice, lime peel and lime juice.

Pour the water into the Instant Pot Insert, and place a trivet with the covered brownie cake tin into the Instant Pot.

Cover your Instant Pot, set the vent to Sealing, select the manual or pressure cook button, select high pressure and set the timer to 30 minutes.

When done allow the pot to undergo natural pressure release for 15 mins

Cool 30 mins. Refrigerate at least 4 hours to chill. Spread whipped topping over chilled cake. Sprinkle with additional lemon and lime peel if desired. Using a serving spatula and a knife to help slide pieces off carefully,

Serve and enjoy

Nutrition Facts

Calories 453, Total Fat 37.4g, Saturated Fat 28.1g, Cholesterol 327mg , Sodium 142mg, Total Carbohydrate 16.6g, Dietary Fiber 2.9g , Total Sugars 13.5g, Protein 14g

Vanilla Pudding

Prep time: 25 min Cooking Time: 15 min serve: 2

Ingredients

1 tablespoon maple syrup

1 tablespoon corn starch

1/8 teaspoon salt

2 cups coconut milk

1 large egg yolks

½ tablespoon unsalted butter

1 teaspoon pure vanilla extract

Instructions

In an Instant Pot, combine maple syrup, corn-starch, salt, coconut milk, and egg yolks. Cover your Instant Pot, set the vent to Sealing, select the manual or pressure cook button, select high pressure and set the timer to 5 minutes.

When done allow the pot to undergo natural pressure release for 15 mins

About 8-10 minutes. Note: It will thicken more as it cools.

Place a fine mesh strainer over a large heatproof bowl. Pour the mixture through the strainer and into the bowl.

Transfer the pudding from the large bowl or into individual serving bowls.

Cool slightly, then cover with plastic wrap. Refrigerate for several hours or until chilled.

Nutrition Facts

Calories 686, Total Fat 62.4g, Saturated Fat 53.4g, Cholesterol 113mg, Sodium 209mg, Total

Carbohydrate 25.1g, Dietary Fiber 5.3g, Total Sugars 14.3g, Protein 6.9g

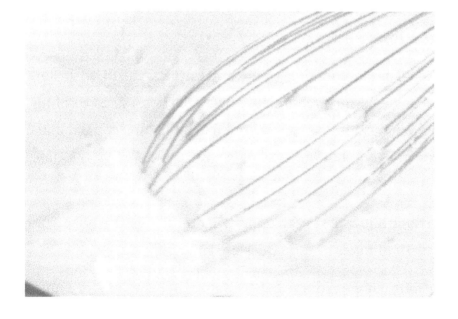

Quick Cherry Crisp

Prep time: 25 min Cooking Time: 25 min serve: 2

Ingredients

¼ cup honey

½ tablespoon corn-starch

2 cups red cherries

½ cup crumbled shortbread cookies

1 tablespoon butter or margarine, melted

1/8 cup chopped almonds, toasted

Ice cream (optional)

Instructions

In a small bowl, combine honey and cornstarch. In an instant pot, sprinkle corn-starch mixture over cherries; stir to combine. Cover your Instant Pot, set the vent to Sealing, select the manual or pressure cook button, select high pressure and set the timer to 2 minutes.

When done allow the pot to undergo natural pressure release for 15 mins 10 minutes or until thickened and bubbly.

Meanwhile, in a medium bowl, thoroughly combine crumbled cookies, butter, and nuts

Divide cherry mixture among four dessert dishes. Sprinkle cookie mixture over cherry mixture. If desired, serve with ice cream.

Nutrition Facts

Calories 241, Total Fat 8.7g, Saturated Fat 3.9g, Cholesterol 15mg, Sodium 43mg, Total Carbohydrate

38.4g, Dietary Fiber 0.8g, Total Sugars 35.1g, Protein 1.5g

Chocolate Chip Cheesecake

Prep time: 25 min Cooking Time: 25 min serve: 2

Ingredients

½ cup graham cracker crumbs

1 tablespoon honey

½ cup unsweetened cocoa powder

½ cup butter, melted

½ cup cream cheese

1 cup sweetened condensed milk

1 egg

1 teaspoon vanilla extract

½ cup mini semi-sweet chocolate chips

1 teaspoon coconut flour

Instructions

Mix graham cracker crumbs, honey, butter and cocoa. Press onto bottom and up the sides of a 9 inch spring form pan. Set crust aside.

Beat cream cheese until smooth. Gradually add sweetened condensed milk; beat well. Add vanilla and egg, and beat on medium speed until smooth. Toss 1/3 of the miniature chocolate chips with the 1 teaspoon coconut flour to coat (this keeps them from sinking to the bottom of the cake). Mix into cheese mixture. Pour into prepared crust. Sprinkle top with remaining chocolate chips.

Pour the water into the Instant Pot Insert, and place a trivet with the covered brownie cake tin into the Instant Pot.

Cover your Instant Pot, set the vent to Sealing, select the manual or pressure cook button, select high pressure and set the timer to 30 minutes.

When done allow the pot to undergo natural pressure release for 15 mins.

Refrigerate before removing sides of pan. Keep cake refrigerated until time to serve.

Nutrition Facts

Calories 418, Total Fat 43.3g, Saturated Fat 26.4g, Cholesterol 160mg, Sodium 458mg, Total Carbohydrate 61.5g, Dietary Fiber 4.3g, Total Sugars 48.4g, Protein 12.7g

Peanut Butter Fudge

Prep time: 25 min Cooking Time: 25 min serve: 2

Ingredients

1 tablespoon honey

1/8 cup coconut milk

½ cup marshmallow crème

1 cups peanut butter

Instructions

In Instant Pot Select Sauté. Add coconut milk and honey. Cover your Instant Pot, set the vent to Sealing, select the manual or pressure cook button, select high pressure and set the timer to 3 minutes.

When done allow the pot to undergo natural pressure release for 15 mins.

Immediately stir in the marshmallow crème and peanut butter.

Pour and spread into a 9x9-inch glass baking dish. Cool completely before cutting into squares and serving.

Nutrition Facts

Calories 480, Total Fat 34.2g, Saturated Fat 8.4g, Cholesterol 0mg0%, Sodium 298mg, Total Carbohydrate 17.5g, Dietary Fiber 4g, Total Sugars 10.6g, Protein 16.3g

Matcha Avocado Pancakes

Preparation Time: 10 minutes Cooking Time: 5 min Servings: 6

Ingredients:

1cup Almond Flour

1 medium-sized Avocado, mashed   1 cup Coconut Milk 1 tbsp Matcha Powder ½ tsp Baking Soda ¼ tsp Salt

Directions:

Mix all Ingredients into a batter. Add water, a tablespoon at a time, to thin out the mixture if needed. Lightly oil a nonstick pan. Scoop approximately 1/3 cup of the batter and cook over medium heat until bubbly on the surface(about 2-3 minutes). Flip the pancake over and cook for another minute.

Nutmeg Pears Small Balls

Prep time: 05 min Cooking Time: 30 min serve: 2

Ingredients

8 oz crescent rolls

1 small pears peeled, cored and cut into 8 wedges

1 tablespoon coconut oil

1/8 cup honey

¼ teaspoon vanilla extract

½ teaspoon ground nutmeg

Pinch ground cardamom

¼ cup red wine

Instructions

Open crescent rolls and separate into 2 triangles. Roll each wedge of pears in 1 crescent roll.

Add coconut oil to the Instant Pot. Use the display panel to select the Saute function.

When coconut oil is about Half melted, turn off the pot by selecting Cancel.

Add honey, vanilla and spices and stir until fully melted and incorporated. Add red wine and stir to combine.

Add dumplings in a single layer, then secure the lid, making sure the vent is closed.

Use the display panel, select the Manual or Pressure Cook function. Use the + /- keys and program the Instant Pot for 10 minutes.

When the time is up, let the pressure naturally release until the pin drops (for 15 minutes, whichever comes first).

Open the pot and let the dumplings cool and set for 3-5 minutes.

Remove dumplings and serve topped with any juices remaining in the pot.

Nutrition Facts

Calories 376, Total Fat 8.9g, Saturated Fat 6.4g, Cholesterol 1mg, Sodium 155mg, Total Carbohydrate

44g, Dietary Fiber 2.9g, Total Sugars 26.2g, Protein 3.5g

Blueberry Milkshakes

Prep time: 05 min Cooking Time: 02 min serve: 2

Ingredients

1 cup whole fat milk

1-1/2 tablespoons maple syrup

½ teaspoon vanilla extract

2 cups blueberries

Instructions

Seat glass pitcher on the base of the Instant Pot Ace.

Add milk, maple syrup, vanilla extract and blueberries.

Secure and lock lid.

Choose the Smoothie program (1:38 minutes).

Serve immediately.

Nutrition Facts

Calories 161, Total Fat 0.5g, Saturated Fat 0g, Cholesterol 3mg, Sodium 62mg, Total Carbohydrate

33.8g, Dietary Fiber 3.5g , Total Sugars 26.5g, Protein 5.6g

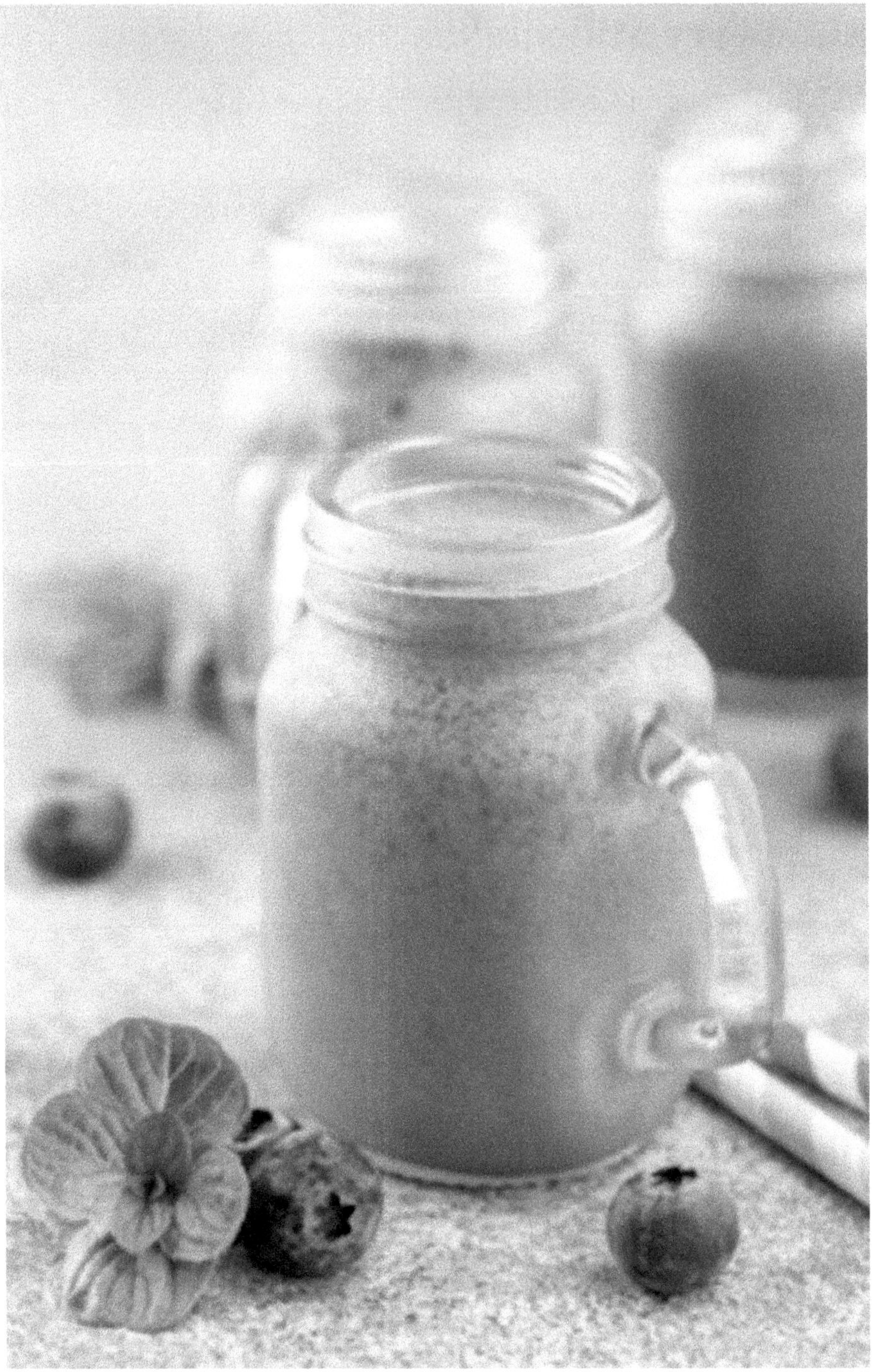

Lava Cakes

Prep time:20 min Cooking Time: 30min serve: 2

Ingredients

¼ cup coconut oil

¼ cup chocolate chopped

½ cup coconut sugar

2 large eggs at room temperature

1 large egg yolk at room temperature

3 tablespoons coconut flour

Pinch salt

½ cup water

Instructions

Put the coconut oil and chocolate in a large, microwave-safe bowl. Microwave on high in 10-second bursts, stirring well after each, until a little over half of the butter has melted. Remove from the microwave oven and continue stirring until smooth.

Set the chocolate mixture aside and cool to room temperature, stirring occasionally, about 20 minutes.

Stir the coconut sugar into the chocolate mixture until smooth. Stir in the eggs one at a time, ensuring each is well incorporated before adding the next. Stir in the eggs yolk until smooth, then the flour and salt, stirring again until smooth. Divide this mixture evenly among the prepared ramekins. Do not cover the ramekins.

Pour the water in the cooker. Set a trivet in the pot, then stack the 4 ramekins on the trivet. Lock the lid onto the cooker.

Press Pressure cook on Max pressure for 8 minutes with the Keep Warm setting off.

When the machine has finished cooking, turn it off and let its pressure return to normal naturally, about 20 minutes. Unlatch the lid and open the cooker. Transfer the hot ramekins to a wire rack and cool for 15 minutes. Serve warm.

Nutrition Facts

Calories 353, Total Fat 33.6g, Saturated Fat 25.6g, Cholesterol 186mg, Sodium 158mg, Total Carbohydrate 7g, Dietary Fiber 0.1g, Total Sugars 1.9g, Protein 6.8g

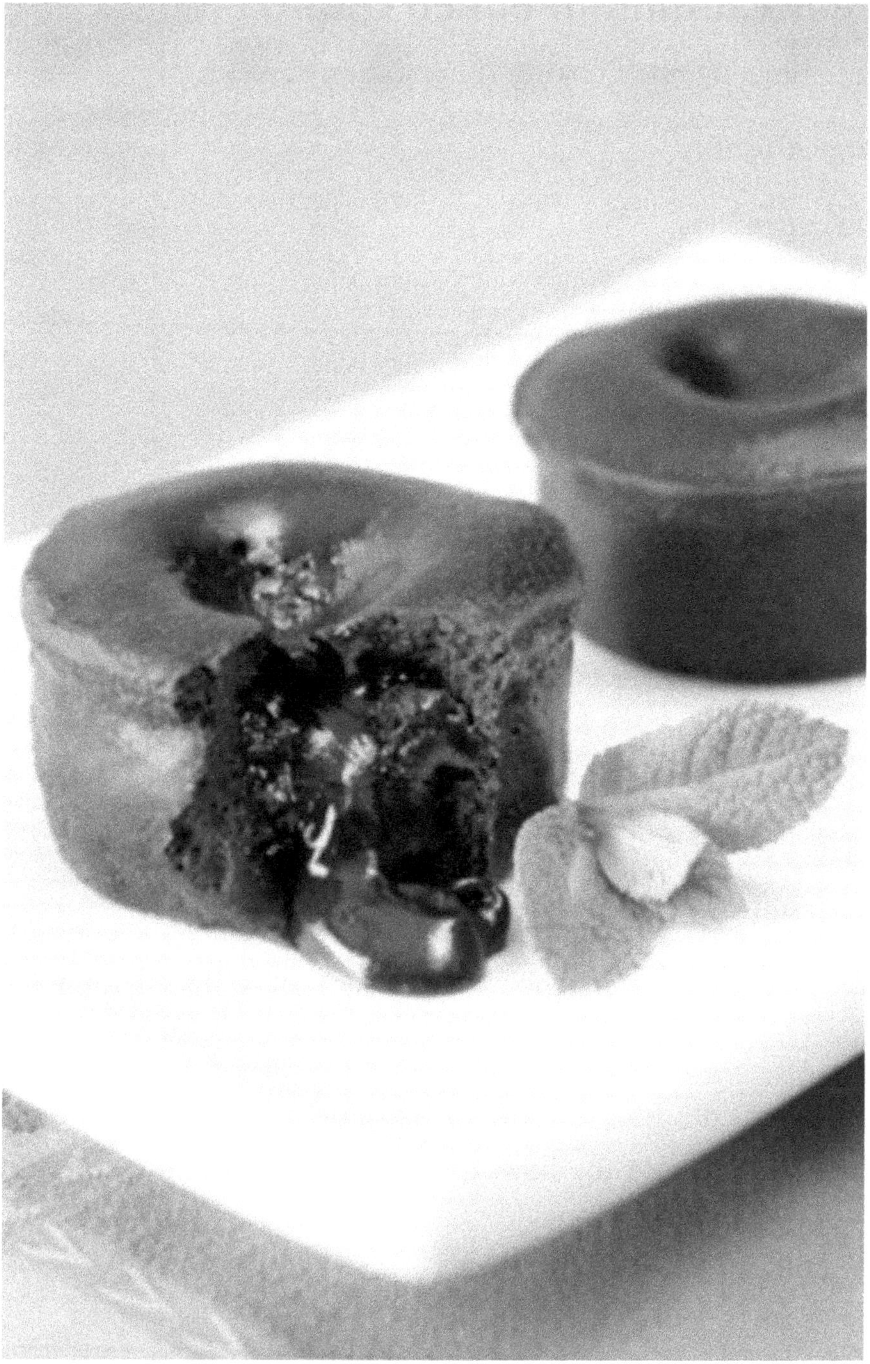

Pear Cinnamon Baked Quinoa

Prep time: 05 min Cooking Time: 10 min Serve: 2

Ingredients

1/2 cup quinoa

1/3 cup coconut milk

1/4 teaspoon baking powder

1/4 teaspoon cinnamon

1/2 teaspoon vanilla

1 teaspoon honey

1/4 cup diced pears

2 cups of water

Instructions

Mix all ingredients in a bowl. Mix them well so that all quinoa is moist.

Put 2 cups of water into the Instant Pot and place the trivet on the bottom. Place the bowl in the Instant Pot and lock lid by closing the pressure valve.

Cook at High Pressure for 10 minutes with the Manual setting. When done, open the Instant Pot and let the pressure release naturally. Take the bowl out of the Instant Pot.

Serve hot.

Nutrition Facts

Calories 287, Total Fat 12.2g, Saturated Fat 8.8g, Cholesterol 0mg, Sodium 10mg, Total Carbohydrate

39.2g, Dietary Fiber 5.3g, Total Sugars 8.3g, Protein 7.1g

Keto snickerdoodles

Keto snickerdoodles are easy soft keto cookies with a delicious cinnamon flavor

Prep Time: 15 mins Cook Time: 12 mins Total Time: 27 mins

Ingredients

Dry ingredients

1 1/3 cup Almond Flour

2 tablespoons Coconut Flour

1/3 cup Erythritol - erythritol or monk fruit 1/2 teaspoon Baking soda

1/2 teaspoon Xanthan gum

Liquid ingredients

1/4 cup Coconut oil or melted butter

1/4 cup Unsweetened vanilla almond milk at room temperature
1 teaspoon Vanilla essence

1 teaspoon Apple cider vinegar Cinnamon coating

2 teaspoons Ground cinnamon

3 tablespoons Erythritol - erythritol or monk fruit

Instructions

In a large mixing bowl, whisk together all the dry ingredients: almond flour, coconut flour, sweetener, baking soda, xanthan gum.

Pour the melted coconut, unsweetened almond milk (at room temperature or it will solidify the coconut oil), vanilla and apple cider vinegar.

Combine with a spoon at first, then use your hands to knead the dough and form a consistent cookie dough ball. Set aside in the bowl, at room temperature, while you prepare the cinnamon coating.

In a separate bowl, whisk together ground cinnamon and sugar-free crystal sweetener of your choice.

Shape 16 small cookie dough balls. I am using a small mechanical cookie dough scoop to make cookies of the same size and same carb count.

Roll each cookie dough balls into the cinnamon sugar-free sugar, rolling the balls in your hands to stick the coating to the balls. Place each cookie ball onto a baking tray covered with parchment paper, leaving 1 cm space between each cookie.

Flatten the snickerdoodle cookie with a spatula until the sides crack and the thickness is similar to a regular snickerdoodle cookie. These cookies won't expand while baking that is why it is important to shape/flatten them before baking.

Repeat for the following cookies.

Bake cookies at 180°C/355°F for 15-18 minutes or until the sides are slightly golden brown, don't overbake are they won't be as soft.

Remove from the oven and cool down 5 minutes on the baking tray before transferring on a cooling rack. Slide a spatula under each cookie to gently transfer them onto a cooling rack without breaking.

The cookie are soft at first when out of the oven, they will harden and reach their best texture at room temperature, about 1 hour cool down required.

Nutrition Info

Calories 76 Calories from Fat 43 Fat 4.8g Carbohydrates 2.2g Fiber 0.8g Sugar 0.5g1% Protein 1.2g

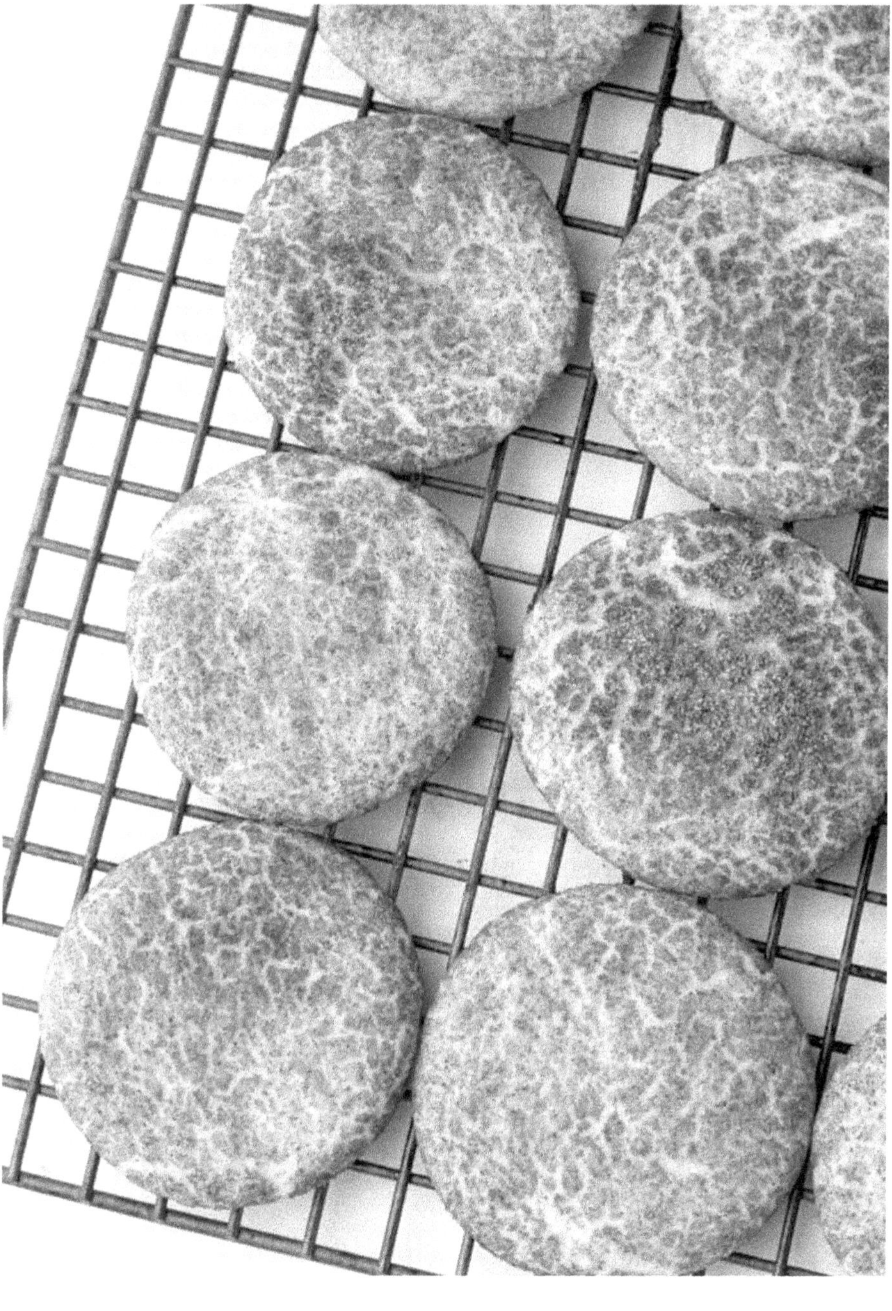

Low carb shortbread cookies with almond flour

Those low carb shortbread cookies with almond flour are easy 5 ingredients healthy shortbread cookies perfect for the holidays.

Prep Time: 10 mins Cook Time: 10 mins Total Time: 20 mins

Ingredients

1 1/3 cup Almond Flour 1/4 cup erythritol

1/4 cup Soft Unsalted Butter at room temperature for 3 hours

1/2 teaspoon Vanilla essence

1/8 teaspoon salt Chocolate decoration - optional

1 oz Sugar-free Chocolate Chips 1/2 teaspoon Coconut oil

Instructions

Preheat oven to 356 F (180C).

Cover a baking sheet with parchment paper. Set aside.

Mix all of the ingredients together until it forms a cookie crumble - about 1 minute. You can use a stand mixer with a hook attachment or an electric mixer.

Gather the cookie crumble with your hands to form a cookie ball.

Refrigerate 10 minutes in a bowl.

Remove from the fridge, scoop 1 teaspoon of dough onto the prepared baking sheet leaving a thumb space between each cookie. You can also roll the dough in your hands and form balls. Then use a fork to slightly flatten the cookie.

Bake your shortbread cookies for 8 -11 minutes or until they start to be golden brown on the top.

Remove from the oven and cool down for 10 minutes on the baking sheet before transferring them to a cooling cookie rack to cool completely before decorating.

Add the sugar free chocolate and coconut oil into a saucepan. Under medium heat, stir and melt the chocolate.

Use a scoop to drizzle a bit of chocolate on some (or all) cookies.

Store the cookies in a cookie jar up to 3 weeks.

Nutrition Info

Calories 81 Calories from Fat 68 Fat 7.5g Carbohydrates 1.9g Fiber 1g Sugar 0.4g Protein 2.1g

Keto Egg Fast Snickerdoodle Crepes

A delicious keto egg fast crepe recipe based on the popular snickerdoodle cookie! Low carb, keto, lchf, egg fast, and Atkins diet friendly recipe.

Servings: Approximately 4 servings

Ingredients

For the crepes:

6 eggs

5 oz cream cheese, softened 1 tsp cinnamon

1 Tbsp granulated sugar substitute (Splenda, Swerve, Ideal, etc.)

butter for frying

For the filling:

8 Tbsp butter, softened

1/3 cup granulated sugar substitute 1 Tbsp (or more) cinnamon

Instructions

Blend all of the crepe ingredients (except the butter) together in a blender or magic bullet until smooth. Let the batter rest for 5 minutes.

Heat butter in a nonstick pan on medium heat until sizzling. Pour enough batter into the pan to form a 6 inch crepe. Cook for about 2 minutes, then flip and cook for an additional minute.

Remove and stack on a warm plate. You should end up with about 8 crepes.

Meanwhile, mix your sweetener and cinnamon in a small bowl or baggie until combined.

Stir half of the mixture into your softened butter until smooth. To serve, spread 1 Tbsp of the butter mixture onto the center of your crepe.

Roll up and sprinkle with about 1 tsp of additional sweetener/cinnamon mixture.

Nutrition Info

Serving Size: 2 crepes, 2 Tbsp filling Calories: 434

Fat: 42g Carbohydrates: 2g net Protein: 12g

Sun Dried Tomato Pesto Mug Cake

Servings 1 Sun Dried Tomato Pesto Mug Cake

Ingredients

Base

1 large egg

2 tablespoons butter

2 tablespoons almond flour

½ teaspoon baking powder

5 teaspoons sun dried tomato pesto 1 tablespoon almond flour

Pinch salt

Instructions

Get your mug ready! Add 1 Large Egg, 3 Tbsp. Honeyville Almond Flour, 2 Tbsp. of Room Temperature Butter, 5 tsp. Sun Dried Tomato Pesto, 1/2 tsp. Baking Powder and a pinch of salt.

Mix everything together well.

Microwave this for 75 seconds on high (power level 10).

Then, lightly slam your mug against a plate so that it comes out. Top with extra cheese sun dried tomato and a small wedge of fresh tomato!

Nutrition Info

429 Calories 40.45g Fats 5.32g Net Carbs 12.34g Protein

Keto Cannoli Stuffed Crepes

These Keto Cannoli Stuffed Crepes are perfect for any special occasion breakfast or brunch! Tastes like you're cheating, but they are low carb, gluten free, grain free, Atkins, and nut free too!

Prep Time: 15 minutes Cook Time: 20 minutes Total Time: 35 minutes Servings: 4 servings

Ingredients

For the crepes:

8 ounces cream cheese, softened

8 eggs

1/2 teaspoon ground cinnamon

1 tablespoon granulated erythritol sweetener 2 tablespoons butter, for the pan

For the cannoli filling:

6 ounces mascarpone cheese, softened 1 cup whole milk ricotta cheese

1/2 teaspoon lemon zest

1/2 teaspoon ground cinnamon

1/4 teaspoon unsweetened vanilla extract 1/4 cup powdered erythritol sweetener

For the optional chocolate drizzle (not included in Nutrition Info:)

3 s☐uares of a Lindt 90% chocolate bar

Instructions

For the crepes:

Combine all of the crepes ingredients in a blender and blend until smooth.

Let the batter rest for 5 minutes and then give it a stir to break up any additional air bubbles.

Heat 1 teaspoon of butter in a 10 inch or larger nonstick saute pan over medium heat.

When the butter is melted and bubbling, pour in about 1/4 cup of batter (you can eyeball it) and if necessary, gently tilt the pan in a circular motion to create a 6-inch (-ish) round crepe.

Cook for two minutes, or until the top is no longer glossy and bubbles have formed almost to the middle of the crepe.

Carefully flip and cook for another 30 seconds. Remove and place on a plate.

Repeat until you have 8 usable crepes.

For the cannoli filling:

Place all of the filling ingredients in a medium-sized bowl and fold gently with a silicone spatula until fully combined.

Spoon the filling into a pastry bag fitted with a large star tube. (If you don't have a pastry bag, use a gallon sized plastic bag with the corner cut out to create a 1 inch wide opening.) Alternatively you can just smear it on the crepe with a spoon.

Pipe a line of filling down the center of one crepe.

Fold the right side over the filling, and then the left side over the top to create a roll.

Repeat with the remaining 7 crepes.

Serve immediately or store, covered, in the refrigerator for up to 3 days.

For the optional chocolate drizzle (not included in Nutrition Info):

Just before serving the crepes, place the s□uares of chocolate in a small bowl.

Microwave on high, uncovered, for 30 seconds. Stir. If   not melted, microwave for another 10 seconds. Stir.

Scrape the melted chocolate into a small plastic bag and cut a tiny bit of one bottom corner off.

Gently s☐ueeze the bag to drizzle the chocolate over the crepes.

Nutrition Info

Serving Size: 2 stuffed crepes Calories: 478 Fat: 42g Carbohydrates: 4g Fiber: 0g Protein: 16g

Peanut Butter Granola Balls

Peanut Butter Granola Balls or Keto energy bites are healthy, no bake, vegan, peanut butter chia seeds and almonds balls with sugar free chocolate chips.

Prep Time: 10 mins Total Time: 20 mins

Servings: 12 granola balls

Ingredients

Dry ingredients

1 cup Sliced almonds 1/4 cup Pumpkin seeds 1 tablespoon Chia seeds

2 tablespoon Flaxseed meal

1/4 cup Unsweetened desiccated Coconut 1/4 teaspoon Salt

1/4 cup Sugar-free Chocolate Chips or dark chocolate chips

>85% cocoa or cocoa nibs Li☐uid ingredients

1/2 cup Natural Peanut butter smooth, unsalted

1/4 cup Sugar-free flavored maple syrup or liquid sweetener of choice

Chcoolate drizzle

1/4 cup Sugar-free Chocolate Chips 1/2 teaspoon Coconut oil

Instructions

In a large mixing bowl add all the dry ingredients, stir to combine, set aside. Note: you can add the chocolate chips now and they will melt in the next step giving a chocolate peanut butter flavor to the ball or you can choose to add the chocolate chips after step 3 to keep the crunchy chocolate chips bites in the balls.

In a small bowl, add the li☐uid ingredients: peanut butter and sugar-free li☐uid sweetener, microwave 45 seconds. This step will soften the peanut butter making it easier to combine with the dry ingredients. Don't over-warm.

Pour the li☐uid ingredients onto the dry ingredients, combine using a spatula until it forms a sticky batter that you can easily shape into granola balls. If you didn't add the chocolate chips in step 1, stir in now.

Slightly grease your hands with coconut oil, grab some dough and roll the granola balls. I recommend a 'golf ball' size to make 12 granola balls in total with this batter.

Roll the prepared granola balls in extra sliced almonds if you like to add some crunch on the sides. Place the granola ball on a plate that you have covered with parchment paper - this prevents the ball from sticking to the plate.

Repeat the rolling process until you form 12 granola balls. Place the plate in the freezer for 10 minutes to firm up the granola balls. Meanwhile melt the extra chocolate chips with coconut oil.

Remove the plate from the freezer, drizzle some melted chocolate on top of each granola ball. Place the plate in the freezer again for 5 minutes to set the chocolate drizzle.

Store up to 3 weeks in the fridge in an airtight container or up to 10 days in the pantry in a cookie jar.

Nutrition Info

Calories 145 Calories from Fat 107 Fat 11.9g Carbohydrates 7.5g Fiber 3.3g Sugar 1.5g Protein 5.3g

Chocolate Peanut Butter Chia Seed Pudding

Ground chia seed pudding with Almond milk is a smooth chocolate peanut butter healthy dessert or breakfast.

Prep Time: 10 mins Total Time: 1 hr 10 mins

Servings: 6 pudding

Ingredients

2/3 cup Chia seeds whole, black or white or 1 cup ground chia seeds

3 tablespoons unsweetened cocoa powder

2 cups unsweetened Almond Breeze Almond Milk (or original if not keto)

2 tablespoons Natural Peanut butter

1/4 cup Sugar-free flavored maple syrup or any liquid sweetener you like (maple syrup, agave, brown rice syrup) 1/2 teaspoon Vanilla essence

1/4 teaspoon Salt

Instructions

Place the chia seed into a blender and blend for about 20 seconds to form ground chia seeds.

Add all the rest of the ingredients - order doesn't matter.

Blend again for 30 seconds to 1 minute until all the ingredients come together. If it sticks to the sides of the blender, you can stop the blender every 30 seconds, scrape down the side, and repeat until smooth. You can't over-process it!

Taste and adjust texture and sweetness. Add more almond milk, 1 tablespoon at a time for a runnier pudding. This may be useful if you replace the sugar-free li□uid sweetener with crystal sweetener (erythritol or monk fruit sugar).

Transfer into ramekin or serving jar. Decorate with a dollop of fresh peanut butter, drizzle melted sugar-free dark chocolate and chopped peanuts.

Enjoy immediately or refrigerate for at least 1 hour for a fresher pudding.

Store for up to 4 days in the fridge in an airtight container.

Nutrition Info

Calories 203 Calories from Fat 111 Fat 12.3g19%

Carbohydrates 24.5g Fiber 19.6g82% Sugar 0.7g1% Protein 6.4g

Milkshake ice pops

Prep:10 mins plus 4 hrs freezing, no cook easy Makes 4

Ingredients

405ml can light condensed milk

1 tsp vanilla bean paste

1 ripe chopped banana

10 strawberries or 3 tbsp chocolate hazelnut spread

Directions:

Pour the light condensed milk into a food processor and add the vanilla bean paste and chopped banana. Whizz until smooth. Add either the strawberries or chocolate hazelnut spread and whizz again.

Divide the mixture between 4 paper cups, cover with foil, then push a lolly stick through the foil lid of each cup until you hit the base. Freeze for 4 hrs or until solid. Will keep in the freezer for 2 months.

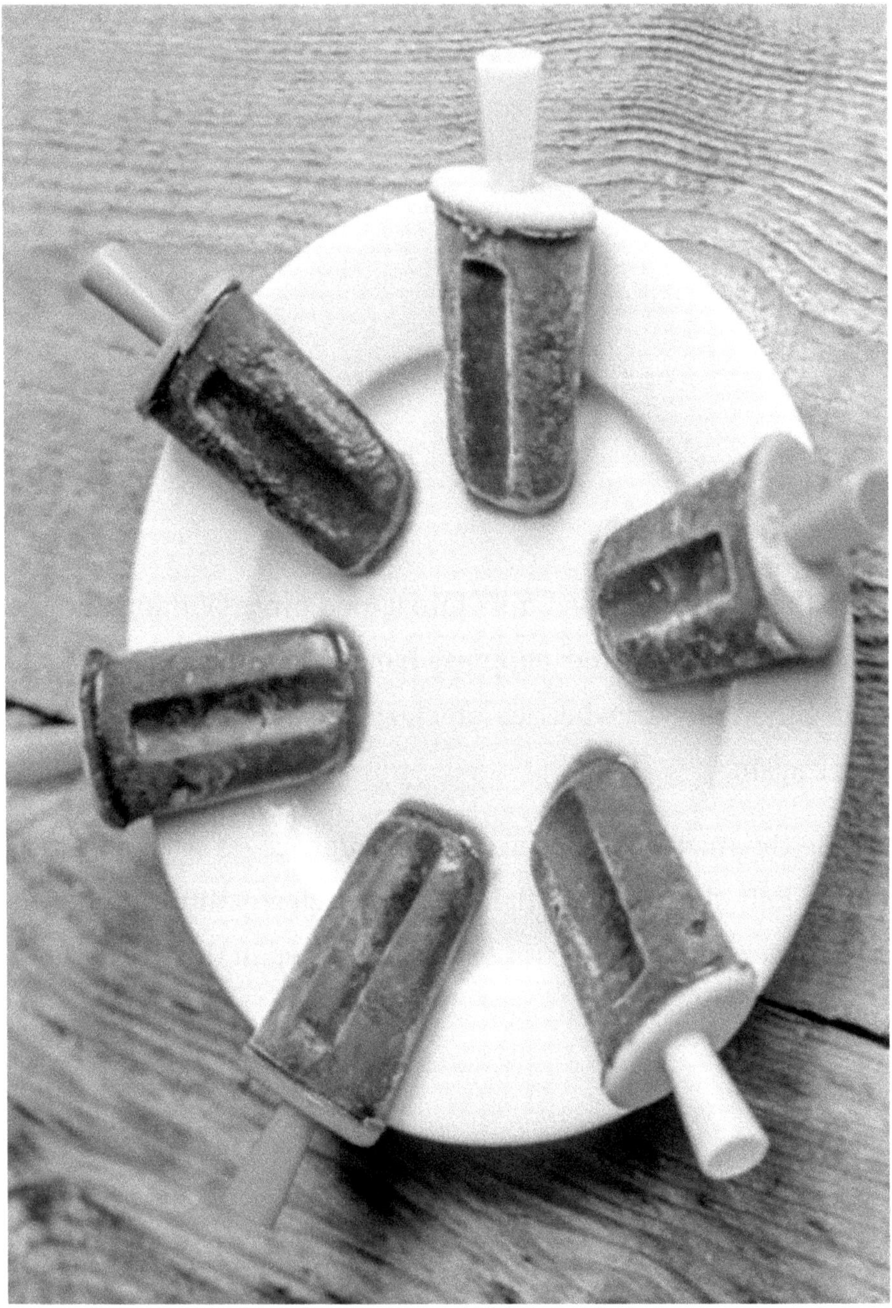

Whisky & pink peppercorn marmalade kit Easy

Ingredients

500g mix of oranges, clementines and lemons

1kg demerara sugar

small pot of pink peppercorns

small bottle of whisky

Optional extras

jam pan muslin

large wooden spoon

small jars and labels (makes about 1kg jam)

To use kit see tip

Directions:

To use the kit:

Write the following instructions on the gift tag:Halve the fruits and squeeze the juices into a large saucepan. Remove all the peel and set aside. Put the flesh in the pan with 1 litre water and boil for 15 mins. Push through a sieve lined with muslin and return the liquid to the pan.

Shred the peel and tip into a heatproof bowl. Add enough water to just cover and microwave for 3-4 mins until soft. Add the peel to the pan, then add the sugar. Boil for 35-45 mins until the marmalade has reached setting point (keep an eye on it so it doesn't bubble over).

Remove from the heat and add 1 tsp pink peppercorns. Allow the mixture to cool a little, then stir in 50ml whisky. Ladle into sterilised jars and seal. Will keep for up to one year.

Simnel muffins

Prep:45 mins - 55 mins easy Makes 12

Ingredients

250g mixed dried fruit

grated zest and juice 1 medium orange

175g softened butter

175g golden caster sugar

3 eggs , beaten

300g self-raising flour

1 tsp mixed spice

½ tsp freshly grated nutmeg

5 tbsp milk

175g marzipan

200g icing sugar

2 tbsp orange juice for mixing

mini eggs

Directions:

Tip the fruit into a bowl, add the zest and juice and microwave on medium for 2 minutes (or leave to soak for 1 hour). Line 12 deep muffin tins with paper muffin cases.

Preheat the oven to fan 180C/ 160C/gas

Beat the butter, sugar, eggs, flour, spices and milk until light and fluffy (about 3-5 minutes) – use a wooden spoon or hand held mixer. Stir the fruit in well. Half fill the muffin cases with the mixture. Divide the marzipan into 12 equal pieces, roll into balls, then flatten with your thumb to the size of the muffin cases. Put one into each muffin case and spoon the rest of the mixture over it. Bake for 25-30 minutes, until risen, golden and firm to the touch. Leave to cool.

Beat together the icing sugar and orange juice to make icing thick enough to coat the back of a wooden spoon. Drizzle over the muffins and top with a cluster of eggs. Leave to set. Best eaten within a day of making.

Prunes Cake

Prep time:20 min Cooking Time: 50min serve: 2

Ingredients

¼ cup vegetable oil

¼ cup honey

1 egg

2 cups coconut flour

½ teaspoon salt

1 teaspoon baking powder

1 cup coconut milk

1 teaspoon vanilla extract

¼ teaspoon almond extract

2 cups chopped prunes, divided

¼ cup water

1 tablespoon lemon juice

Instructions

Spray two 8-inch round cake pans with vegetable oil spray.

In a medium bowl, sift together coconut flour, salt and baking powder. Set aside.

In a large mixing bowl, making cream add vegetable oil with the honey until fluffy. Add egg and beat well. Add flour mixture coconut milk. Fold in vanilla and almond extracts and 1 cup chopped prunes.

Pour water into Instant Pot. Place wire trivet into the bottom of the pot and set the pan on top. Place lid on pot and lock into place to seal. Pressure Cook or Manual on High Pressure for 30 minutes. Let sit 10 minutes. Use Quick Pressure Release. Keep cake aside.

To make the filling: In an Instant pot, combine reaming chopped prunes, honey, and water and lemon juice. Close the lid of Instant pot, Pressure Cook or Manual on High Pressure for 20 minutes. Let sit 10 minutes. Use Quick Pressure Release. Spread thinly between cooled cake layers and on top.

Nutrition Facts

Calories 316, Total Fat 23.9g, Saturated Fat 12.7g, Cholesterol 33mg, Sodium 256mg, Total Carbohydrate 77.2g, Dietary Fiber 4.9g, Total Sugars 28.9g, Protein 8.2g

Butternut squash Almond Cookies

Prep time: 40 min Cooking Time: 25 min serve: 2

Ingredients

1 cup butter, soften

¼ cup honey

1 egg, beaten

¼ teaspoon vanilla extract

1 cup butternut squash. puree

2 cups coconut flour

1 teaspoon baking powder

1 teaspoon baking soda

¼ teaspoon salt

1 teaspoon ground nutmeg

¼ cup walnuts

Instructions

Line the Instant Pot with parchment paper and spray with nonstick coconut oil spray. Set aside.

Cream together the butter and honey.

Beat together the egg, vanilla and butternut squash puree.

Sift together the coconut flour, baking powder, baking soda, salt and nutmeg; combine with butternut squash mixture and stir in almond.

Add the cookie dough to the prepared Instant pot. Using a rubber spatula, spread and press the dough into the bottom of the pot, making sure to cover the bottom completely and filling in any gaps.

Cover and lock the lid, but leave the steam release handle in the Venting position. Select High pressure and set the cook time for 15 min. When the cook time is complete, press Cancel to turn off the pot.

Open the lid and carefully transfer the inner pot with the cookie to a cooling rack. Allow the cookie to cool in the pot for a minimum of 30 minutes or until it reaches room temperature.

Nutrition Facts

Calories 193, Total Fat 17.4g, Saturated Fat 10g, Cholesterol 54mg, Sodium 270mg, Total Carbohydrate 8.1g, Dietary Fiber 0.8g , Total Sugars 6.6g, Protein 1.5g

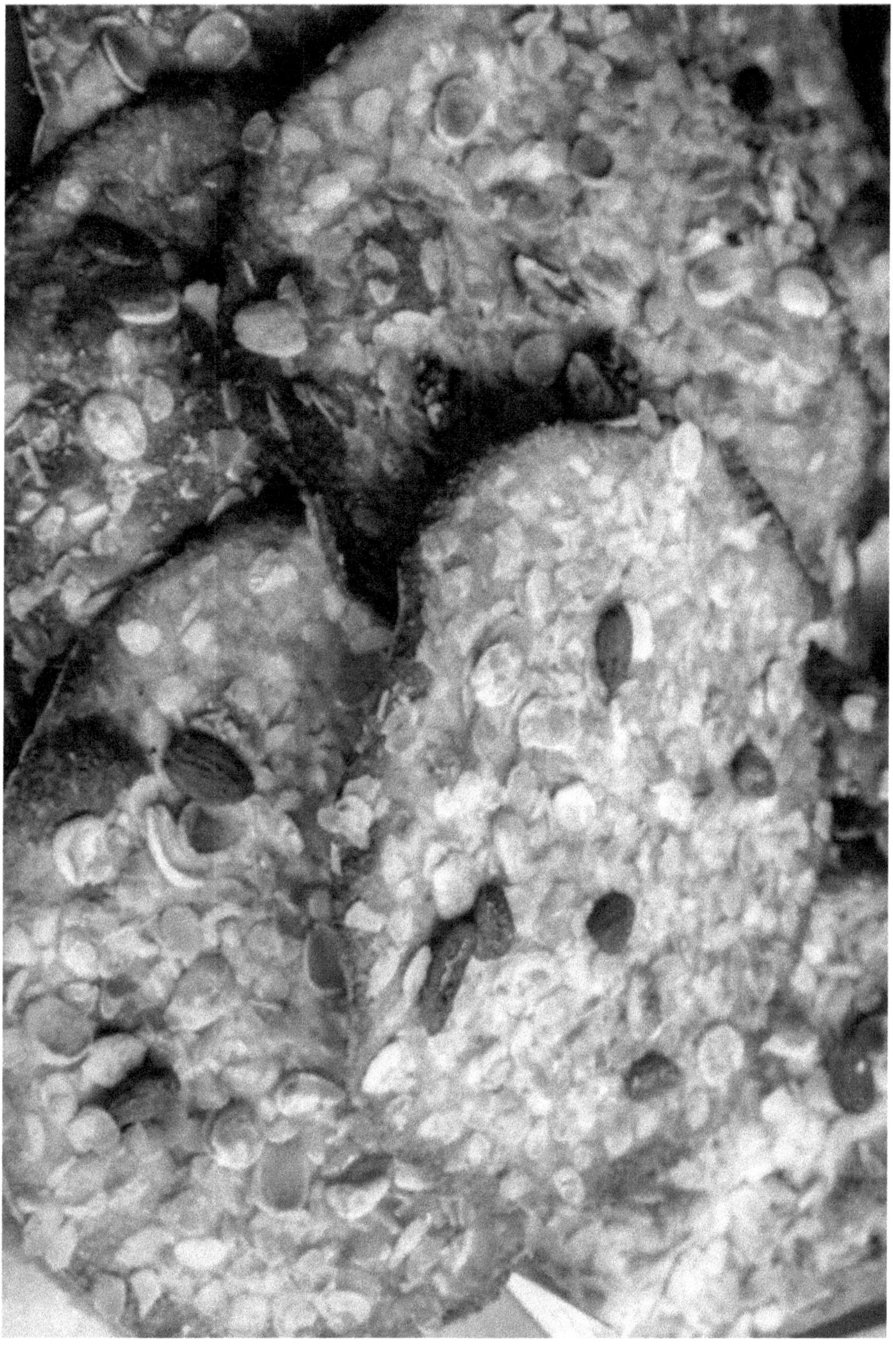

Blackberries Compote

Prep time: 15 min Cooking Time: 20 min serve: 2

Ingredients

4 cups fresh blackberries

¼ cup maple syrup

1 teaspoon freshly squeezed lemon juice

1 teaspoon orange juice

Instructions

Wash all the blackberries.

Add the blackberries and maple syrup to the Instant Pot. Add the lemon juice and orange juice

Lock the lid in place. Select Pressure Cook or Manual, and adjust the pressure to High and the time to 2 minutes. After cooking, let the pressure release naturally for 10 minutes, then quickly release any remaining pressure.

Unlock the lid. Taste the berries (carefully—they're hot) and adjust the sweetness if necessary.

Nutrition Facts

Calories 250, Total Fat 1.5g, Saturated Fat 0.1g, Cholesterol 0mg, Sodium 7mg, Total Carbohydrate

54.4g, Dietary Fiber 15.3g , Total Sugars 37.5g, Protein 4g

Raspberry-Vanilla Barley Pudding

Prep time: 10 min Cooking Time: 45 min serve: 2

Ingredients

1 cup water

1 cup coconut milk

1 tablespoon honey

½ cup raspberries fresh

½ cup barley

¼ teaspoon nutmeg

¼ teaspoon vanilla

½ cup coconut cream

Instructions

Select Sauté on the Instant Pot and adjust to normal. Add the coconut milk, water, honey, to the pot.

Press cancel. Stir in the barley and nutmeg and vanilla into the pot. Secure the lid on the Instant Pot.

Close the pressure-release valve. Select porridge. When cooking is complete, use a natural-release to depressurize.

Remove and Stir in fresh raspberries and cream.

Nutrition Facts

Calories 502,Total Fat 29.9g, Saturated Fat 25.7g, Cholesterol 0mg , Sodium 28mg, Total Carbohydrate

49.3g, Dietary Fiber 10.7g, Total Sugars 13.2g, Protein 8.5g

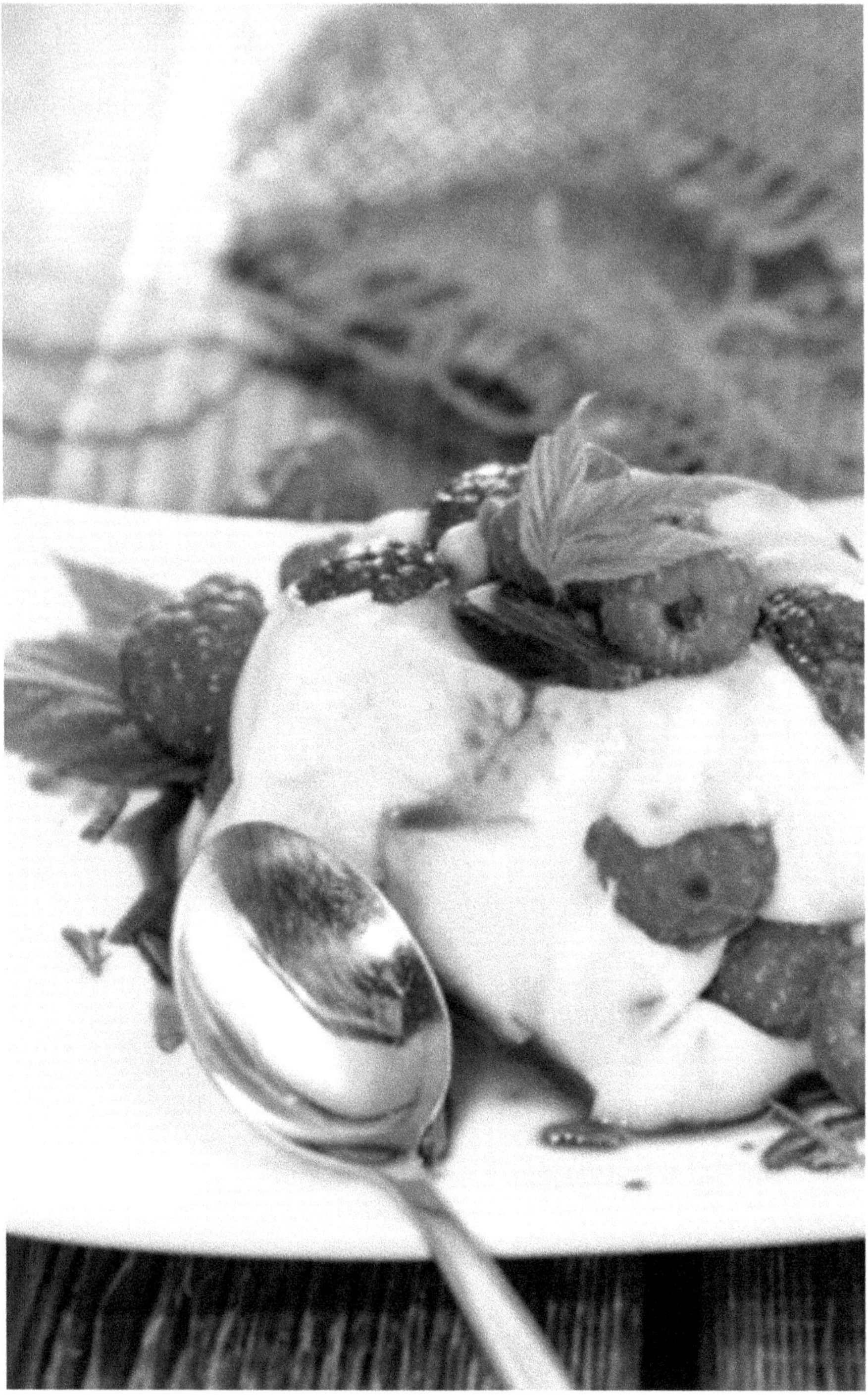

Lightning Source UK Ltd.
Milton Keynes UK
UKHW020638220421
382432UK00010B/566

9 781801 456494